What the NATIONAL INSTITUTE OF DRUG ABUSE *TRIED* TO HIDE

The Medicinal Properties of Cannabis Acknowledged

By Russell Redden

includes
Chapter 9
of
Monograph 14:
"Marihuana Research Findings, 1976"

What the National Institute of Drug Abuse Tried to Hide:
The Medicinal Properties of Cannabis Acknowledged

By Russell Redden

© 2017 By Russell Redden. All Rights Reserved.

Chapter 9 of "Marihuana Research Findings 1976" is reproduced in this work in its entirety, with references.

Released into the Public Domain, and to Congress, 1977.

ISBN-13:
978-1545124826

ISBN-10:
1545124825

What the NATIONAL INSTITUTE OF DRUG ABUSE *TRIED* TO HIDE

The Medicinal Properties of Cannabis Acknowledged

By Russell Redden

includes
Chapter 9
of
Monograph 14:
"Marihuana Research Findings, 1976"

Sections

Introduction..7

Chapter 9: Marihuana Research Findings: 1976:
THERAPEUTIC ASPECTS...11
    The Ancient Lore...13
    The Middle Period...16
    The Current Period..18
    Intraocular Pressure (IOP) Reduction....................19
    Bronchodilation...20
    Anticonvulsant..22
    Retardation of Tumor Growth................................24
    Antibacterial Activity..25
    Sedative-Hypnotic Action......................................25
    Analgesia..26
    Pre-Anesthetic..28
    Antidepressant..29
    Antinauseant, Antiemetic and Appetite Enhancer......................30
    Treatment of Alcohol and Drug Dependence............30
    The Synthetics..31
    Mechanism of Therapeutic Action..........................31
    Conclusion to Monograph Chapter.........................32
    References..33

Conclusion..43

INTRODUCTION

For the past four decades, the placement of Marijuana in Schedule 1 of the Controlled Substances Act of 1970 has hindered research. This is a declaration by the Government that this substance has no medicinal value. This determination puts researchers through a maze of regulations, in order to get permission to test this drug on a human being.

At the time this drug was scheduled, there was a large volume of evidence that proved marijuana has medical value. This evidence was presented in a chapter of "Marihuana Research Findings 1976." This data—available to the public, and all elected representatives—presented the history of the medical use of Cannabis, and listed several serious conditions that could possibly be treated, with references to the clinical evidence.

The link to Research Monograph 14 was conspicuously missing from the list of all monographs on the National Institute of Drug Abuse's web site:

- Monograph 18: **Behavioral Tolerance: Research and Treatment Implications**
- Monograph 4: **Narcotic Antagonists: The search for Long-Acting Preparations**
- Monograph 3: **Aminergic Hypotheses of Behavior: Reality or Cliche?**

1977

- Monograph 16: **The Epidemiology of Heroin and Other Narcotics**
- Monograph 15: **Review of Inhalants: Euphoria to Dysfunction**
- Monograph 13: **Cocaine: 1977**
- Monograph 12: **Psychodynamics of Drug Dependence**
- Monograph 11: **Drugs and Driving**
- Monograph 10: **The Epidemiology of Drug Abuse: Current Issues**

1976

- Monograph 9: **Narcotic Antagonists: Naltrexone**
- Monograph 8: **Rx :3 x /Week Laam Alternative to Methadone**
- Monograph 7: **Cannabinoid Assays in Humans**
- Monograph 6: **Effects of Labeling the "Drug Abuser": An Inquiry**
- Monograph 5: **Young Men and Drugs - A Nationwide Survey**

1975

- Monograph 2: **Operational Definitions in Socio-Behavioral Drug Use Research**
- Monograph 1: **Findings of Drug Abuse Research**

An image of the links to the Monographs on NIDA's web site Monograph 14 (from 1977) is <u>missing</u>

It is obvious why NIDA would remove this link. Research Monograph 14 *admits* to the medicinal properties of marijuana—in contrast with the declaration the Drug Enforcement Agency has made *year* after *year: marijuana has no medicinal properties, and must remain on Schedule 1.*

This has constricted research into the various deadly conditions listed in this research monograph, *including cancer.* I found this Monograph by accident. Although the link to this publication was removed, it was left on the server, according to the monograph number, and could easily be found by "counting up" in the browser to #14. Of course, copies can be purchased from the U.S. Government printing office—but removing the link was an attempt to hide this information from the general public.

This demonstrates the fraud perpetrated on the American Public —by the continued prohibition against marijuana, which is an unwritten crime against the sick—who could benefit from drugs made from this plant, safer than many current prescription drugs with serious side effects.

Russell Redden

Marihuana Research Findings: 1976

**Released 1977
Chapter 9**

THERAPEUTIC ASPECTS

Sidney Cohen, M.D., D.Sc.

While cannabis is one of the most ancient of drugs used for medicinal purposes, this is no reason to expect that it would pass today's stringent tests of efficacy and toxicity. Nor should one summarily dismiss the possibility that cannabis may have some therapeutic utility simply because the plant is currently the subject of socio-political controversy. The controversy makes its impartial evaluation more difficult, but its potential benefits should be studied with the same careful pre-marketing procedures used for other investigational drugs.

Furthermore, if some substantial utility is found, marihuana itself will not be the marketed product; it is a complex mixture of over a dozen cannabinoids, about 30 terpenes, assorted sterols and other substances, most of which do not contribute to a desired therapeutic effect. Even its active cannabinoids can be improved upon for specific indications by synthetic chemists. The benzopyran structure is an unique one, and it can be modified at many positions on the molecule: if the psychological effects are not desired, they can be eliminated; if water solubility or a longer shelf life is preferred, that can be achieved. Although much more testing is needed, there is promise that certain of the pharmacologic actions of cannabis and its derivatives can be helpful for specific conditions.

As we survey those specific indications for which cannabis may be useful, some appear more promising than others. It is now reasonable to believe that intraocular pressure is reduced by cannabis in both normal subjects and in glaucoma patients with ocular hypertension.-9-THC is the most potent agent for this purpose, and when a safe, topically-instilled ophthalmic preparation is developed, it may come to be a helpful medication in the management of some wideangle glaucoma patients. Although satisfactory antiglaucoma preparations are now available, there is a suggestion that an occasional patient responds better to -9-THC than to those drugs currently in use.

Both asthmatics and normal subjects respond with bronchodilation to aerosolized, smoked or oral -9-THC as well as they do to the conventional antiasthmatic medications. A next logical step will be the development of a non-intoxicating pharmaceutical preparation such as an aerosol or a non-intoxicating congener with bronchodilating properties. Marihuana itself, although a bronchodilator, is unsatisfactory because of its direct irritant effect upon pulmonary tissues.

Further studies will determine whether -9-THC is sufficiently useful clinically in ameliorating the anorexia, nausea and vomiting of cancer chemotherapy patients. In such patients, the standard antiemetics are only partially effective, and a superior, new compound would be quite desirable. Patients in such investigations could also be studied to evaluate the appetite enhancing and antianxiety effects of -9-THC.

Except for isolated case reports, no recent work has been reported in which a cannabinoid was employed for the treatment of epilepsy in humans. The animal data are encouraging, but the finding that -9-THC is also a convulsant in certain animal strains requires caution.

Cannabidiol or one of the synthetics may turn out to be the preferred agent in certain convulsive disorders if the animal work can be extrapolated to the convulsant syndromes in humans. In a number of conditions, the evidence of the clinical effectiveness of the cannabinoids remains either preliminary or ambiguous.

These include the utility of -9-THC as an hypnotic, as a treatment for depression and as an antitumor agent. It appears to offer no advantage over existing pre-anesthetic agents. On the basis of available studies, its analgesic efficacy remains in doubt, despite its widespread use in folk medicine for this purpose.

In addition, it would have to compete in the marketplace with existing effective and stable analgesic compounds. No evidence exists that the cannabinoids are superior to available preparations now in use in the detoxification of drug or alcohol dependent persons. The possibility that hemp may have topical antibiotic activity should be pursued.

In addition to the possibility that therapeutic benefits may, one day, accrue, another reason for studying the potential medicinal value of the cannabinoids is the possibility that their mechanisms of action may be different from the currently available medicaments.

In this case, the elucidation of these mechanisms would be even more significant than the mere discovery of another therapeutic agent. A possible explanation for cannabis' precise mode of action is its inhibitory action on prostaglandin synthetase. Adrenergic stimulation has also been noted at certain end organs, a finding which has led to the investigation of the influence of the cannabinoids on various neurotransmitters; no definitive findings have been reported, however.

Recently, a large series of synthetic benzopyrans have been produced by modifying the cannabinoid structure. These or related analogues may come to be the preferred therapeutic substances. They have been designed to provide a selective action either with or without the psychic effects of cannabis. Some of the synthetic benzopyrans are water soluble, permitting more reliable gastrointestinal absorption and making parenteral administration less difficult.

A promising start has been made in the scientific exploration of the therapeutic potential of the cannabinoids although much more work is needed before any compound will be approved for general medical use for any indication.

A noteworthy effort in assessing the therapeutic potential of marihuana and its constituents was made at the first conference assembled for that purpose during November, 1975 at the Asilomar Conference Center, Monterey, California. Sponsored by the National Institute on Drug Abuse (NIDA), the conference included 28 papers related to preclinical or clinical therapeutics (Cohen & Stillman,1976).

THE ANCIENT LORE

The use of cannabis for purposes of healing predates recorded history. The earliest written reference is found in the 15th century B.C. Chinese Pharmacopeia, the Rh-Ya (Emboden, 1972).

Cannabis had many uses as a medicinal herb in China; these are mentioned in the first or second century A.D. Pen Ts'oo Ching (Rubin, 1976) and are based upon traditions passed down from prehistoric times. In this ancient pharmacopeia, a boiled hemp compound given to surgical patients as an anesthetic is described.

From the Chinese plateau, the use of hemp as a folk medicine, ritual potion, condiment and intoxicating agent spread to India, the Middle East and beyond.

Rubin has reviewed the cross-cultural uses of cannabis, some of which are repetitive, but others are unusual. In Viet Nam, for example, cannabis was used to prevent memory loss and mental confusion, to eliminate blood wastes and to treat gynecological and obstetrical problems, such as dysmenorrhea. Allergies and rheumatism were treated by a preparation made by pulverizing roasted cannabis kernels (seeds?) in baby's urine and taking a small glass of the extract three times a day. It was also employed as a cure for falling hair and tapeworm.

In Cambodia, ganja was used for other purposes, such as restoring appetite. Hemp cigarettes, smoked daily, were also supposed to reduce polyps of the nose and relieve asthma. The Cambodians also administered hemp preparations to facilitate contractions during difficult childbirth.

An examination of the multiple, diverse claims made for the therapeutic benefits of cannabis during earlier epochs reveals that many cannot be justified from our current knowledge of its pharmacologic activity. For example, it had a purported effectiveness in cases of leprosy, gonorrhea and arsenic poisoning. The smoke was tried as an enema for strangulated hernia and juice of the leaves was recommended for dandruff, vermin infestation and for a variety of other skin conditions, usually as a lotion or poultice.

On the other hand, some justification can be found for certain of the ancient medical applications. Cannabis was frequently used for painful conditions like neuralgia, dysmenorrhea and toothache.

Because of its analgesic effect, only partially supported by recent research findings, it also found service in minor operations like circumcision and boil lancing. Its relaxant and euphoriant properties may have been exploited in the management of psychological problems, such as melancholia and hysteria.

A number of therapeutic references can be found involving the seeds of Cannabis sativa L. (Grinspoon, 1971). For example, seventh century Scythians inhaled and bathed in the vapors of hemp seeds thrown on hot coals, and "they howled with joy." This apparently euphoriant effect is doubtful, however, since the seeds contain essentially no -9-THC, and are usually discarded when marihuana is "manicured." Whatever joy the Scythians experienced must have been due to the effects of the sauna. Interestingly, the inhalation of hemp vapors remains a popular form of administering cannabis for toothache in parts of the Ukraine, the same region where Scythians once lived.

Earlier and more recent reports about an aphrodisiac property are not as easily evaluated. Much seems to depend upon the mental set of the consumer. If it is taken for that purpose, sexual interest, activity and enjoyment are likely to be enhanced. However, cannabis was also utilized by sexually abstinent Buddhist monks to diminish sex drives and aid in meditation. While marihuana may enhance sensory perception, prolong the subjective experience of time and reduce inhibitions, thus intensifying the sexual experience, it appears to have no direct effect upon sexual drive states (Cohen, 1975). In fact, in view of reports of lowered plasma testosterone levels after chronic, heavy smoking, there remains the possibility that potency could actually be reduced (Kolodny et al., 1976).

One interesting effect of bhang and ganja mentioned in the Report of the Indian Hemp Drugs Commission (1969) and, more recently, in the Jamaican (Rubin & Comitas, 1975) and Colombian field studies (Rubin, 1976), is the assertion that it is a "creator of energy," that it increases staying power, relieves fatigue and acts as a stimulant. The Jamaican report tells of its use as an energizer and motivator to work. Ganja breaks in the Jamaican hinterland seem to be the equivalent of North American coffee breaks. Employers have been known to supply their employees with ganja to get more work out of them. In Colombia, marihuana is smoked by day-laborers and peasants to reduce fatigue and to give "spirit for working." This energizing effect is the principal motivation for use reported by Jamaican working class males and is in sharp contrast to American concerns about the marihuana-induced "amotivational syndrome."

These conflicting effects are probably reflections of the importance of expectations in determining which pharmacologic effects will become manifest.

Rubin (1976) also points out another facet of the preponderant impact of psychophysiologic set over pharmacologic action of a drug like cannabis when taken in moderate dosages. As mentioned above, it is used as a stimulant during the day among unskilled laborers in Jamaica, but is also taken for its sedative effect at night to promote sleep. We should not be confused about this apparent paradox, since we do the same with our most popular intoxicant, alcohol. Americans drink at social gatherings to achieve a stimulating effect and take a nightcap a few hours later to produce drowsiness. This practice is our contribution to the power of expectation in determining drug action.

Cannabis was one of the more important drugs in the Indian Materia Medica at the turn of the century. It was, and still is, widely used in rural areas of the Indian subcontinent for asthma, bronchitis and loss of appetite. Although a bronchodilator action has recently been quite well established (Tashkin et al., 1974; Vachon et al., 1976b), cannabis is likely to be a cause of, rather than a cure for, bronchitis. Its appetite-stimulating activity is confirmed in numerous subjective reports, although no precise mode of action for this effect is known.

THE MIDDLE PERIOD

During the latter half of the 19th century, a resurgent interest in the medical usefulness of the hemp plant developed. Over 100 papers appeared on the subject in the medical journals of the day, some of which are worth citing briefly.

In Calcutta, O'Shaughnessy (1842) administered cannabis to patients with a variety of ailments, including tetanus, rabies, epilepsy and rheumatism. He reported favorably on its anticonvulsant, analgesic and muscle-relaxing properties. His article sparked a flurry of clinical studies, including those of M'Meens (1860), who considered the drug to be a sedative-hypnotic and of value in such diverse disorders as neuralgia, dysmenorrhea, asthma and sciatica. Other favorable papers appeared, including those of Birch (1889) and Mattison (1891) who recommended cannabis enthusiastically for the treatment of morphinism, alcoholism and other addictions. Reynolds (1890) wrote of its value in senile insomnia and in tic doloureux (trigeminal neuralgia). During this same period, Moreau de Tours (1857) used cannabis successfully to treat a variety of psychiatric syndromes, including melancholia and obsessive-compulsive neurosis.

His positive findings in managing mental disorders were confirmed by some investigators, and challenged by others.

Despite these encouraging testimonials, cannabis began to slip into disuse. By the beginning of the 20th century, several factors had combined to account for its neglect by Western medicine:

1) A standardized preparation was not available. Different batches of the plant had widely varying potencies, from essentially inactive to much stronger than the prescriber anticipated.

2) The drug had an unsatisfactory shelf life. Some of the extracts and fluid extracts were practically inert if they were dispensed a few years after they were obtained from the pharmaceutical firm. -9-THC gradually breaks down into inert cannabinol when stored at room temperature and exposed to light and air. The dried leaves of Cannabis sativa L. and its pharmaceutical preparations were quite unreliable after storage, and some of the contradictory clinical results might be explained on this basis.

3) -9-THC is completely insoluble in water and is absorbed across the gastrointestinal mucosa with some difficulty. Therefore, the oral route of administration is not completely reliable. This may be the reason that swallowed -9-THC is two to three times less effective by weight than the smoked drug.

4) By the early 1900's, a series of synthetic, water soluble analgesics and sedatives with a much more stable and predictable pharmacologic

action had begun to appear. This resulted in a diminished need for and use of cannabis and other botanicals.

5) The final blow to interest in marihuana as a therapeutic agent was the Marijuana Tax Act of 1937 which classified the drug as a narcotic. By that year, however, it was essentially no longer prescribed in the United States.

Even after the first synthetic tetrahydrocannabinol, pyrahexyl (Synhexyl), was produced in 1940, it was not widely employed, although it was tried in the treatment of the depressions, the epilepsies and the addictive states. Some work was done with this synthetic by Thompson and Proctor (1967), who treated certain drug withdrawal syndromes with some success. In what may have been the first double blind study with a cannabinoid, Parker and Wrigley (1950) gave pyrahexyl or a placebo to 57 depressed patients, but were unable to demonstrate a significant difference between the experimental and control groups. Later this study was criticized by Grinspoon (1971) for having used an inadequate dosage level. At any rate, both favorable and unfavorable reports with pyrahexyl are to be found in the literature.

The value of these earlier reports is questionable, except perhaps as preliminary clinical explorations. They were usually uncontrolled and impressionistic, and were not carefully designed. Still, they did provide certain clues that were helpful to subsequent investigators.

Between 1950 and 1965, a series of 30 papers on cannabis were published by Czechoslovakian scientists, principally from the Medical Faculty of the Palacky University of Olomouc. Eighteen of the reports[1] dealt with the use of cannabis as a topical antibiotic.

Kabelik et al. (1960) surveyed thousands of plant varieties for their antibiotic activity and reported that more than 500 cases of herpes labialis and ulcerous gingivitis were successfully treated with a hemp salve or spray. Hubacek (1955) used cannabis in otorhinolaryngological conditions including otitis media, chronic sinusitis and tonsilopharyngitis with good results. The Czechoslovakian orthopedists injected cannabis solutions into a few osteomyelitic fistulas with healing results in some cases. An analgesic effect is often mentioned in these papers, as in two cases of second degree burns. The reports are not widely known, nor have they been confirmed, partly due to their publication in journals that are not widely circulated outside of Czechoslovakia.

THE CURRENT PERIOD

[1] Hubacek, 1955; Kabelik, 1955, 1957; Kabelik et al., 1960; Krejci 1950, 1952, 1955, 1958, 1961a, 1961b; Krejci & Heczko, 1958; Krejci et al., 1959; Krejci & Vybiral, 1962; Navratil, 1955; Procek, 1955; Simek, 1955; Sirek, 1955; Soldan, 1955.

The systematic study of the clinical pharmacology of cannabis did not evolve until the last decade. A number of scientific accomplishments and administrative decisions were required before a modern scientific program could develop. These events included:

1) The total synthesis of -9-THC by Mechoulam and Gaoni (1965), permitting the manufacture of sufficient supplies of pure material for investigators.

2) The elucidation of the relationship between the pharmacology of cannabis and -9-THC indicating that the latter was responsible for most of the activity of the whole plant (Mechoulam et al., 1970).

3) The development of a reliable source of uniform, assayed marihuana grown at the University of Mississippi (Quimby et al., 1973) under contract to NIDA.

4) The availability of a reliable quantitative procedure for -9-THC and other cannabinoids.

5) The development of satisfactory controls for obtaining cannabis or a variety of cannabinoids from NIDA for research purposes.

6) A forward plan designed to fund grants and contracts that would clarify the physiologic, pharmacologic and psychologic properties of cannabis.

7) The recent development of assay procedures for the qualitative analysis of cannabinoids in biological fluids (Agurell et al., 1973).

In the overall pharmacological assessment of cannabis, the drug was found to have effects that were potentially therapeutic. The areas of possible therapeutic application can be placed into two general groups: those that utilize the psychologic changes induced by the drug, and those that do not. In the latter instance, the well-known subjective symptoms are often considered undesired side effects by the patient.

The therapeutic uses that do not utilize the mental effects of the drug include intraocular pressure reduction, bronchodilation, anticonvulsant action and tumor growth retardation. Those therapeutic trials that rely on the mental changes include the evaluation of marihuana's effectiveness as a sedative-hypnotic, analgesic, antidepressant, tranquilizer, pre-anesthetic, antinauseant, antiemetic, antianorexiant as well as its utility in the areas of drug and alcohol dependence.

Intraocular Pressure (IOP) Reduction

Hepler and Frank (1971) studied the spectrum of physiologic ocular changes produced by smoking marihuana. Among their early findings was a consistent, dose-related, clinically significant reduction of intraocular pressure (IOP) in normal subjects. The IOP was also reduced with doses of oral -9-THC, -8-THC and, to a much lesser degree, with cannabinol and cannabidiol. Publications by Shapiro (1974), Purnell and Gregg (1975), and Green and Podos (1974) have confirmed the IOP-reducing effect of marihuana and the tetrahydrocannabinols.

Flom et al. (1975) suggested that the lowering of IOP was apparently secondary to a relaxing and euphoriant effect. However, when Hepler gave subjects full doses of diazepam (Valium) blind, he found that the IOP reduction was not significantly different from the effect of a placebo.

Twelve open angle glaucoma patients were studied by the UCLA group (Hepler et al., 1976). In 10 of the 12, impressive reductions in ocular hypertension were achieved. The reduction averaged 30 percent and lasted 4-5 hours. In two instances, however, the smoked marihuana or ingested -9-THC failed to induce a pressure reduction.

The IOP-reducing effects of cannabis appear to be additive to the conventional glaucoma medications. In a preliminary study of a topically applied eye drop preparation of -9-THC in sesame oil, 12 rabbits showed a 40 percent IOP reduction when compared to those treated with sesame oil alone.

Green (1975) and his associates (Green & Kim, 1976, 1973; Green et al., 1976) demonstrated a decrease in the IOP of rabbits given intravenous -9-THC. They postulated that -9-THC interacts with the adrenergic innervation system of the eye; in other words, that -adrenergic blockade would dampen the -9-THC effect. Apparently, ß-adrenergic blockade also partly inhibits the -9-THC effect. The end result of the adrenergic stimulation by -9-THC appears to be a dilation of the efferent blood vessels, modulated by an inhibition of prostaglandin synthetase. Green and Kim (1973) have concluded that the outflow facility may be regulated by adrenergic receptors with -9-THC acting as a vasodilator of the outflow blood vessels of the anterior uvea. There is also the possibility that cannabis acts to constrict afferent episcleral plexus vessels.

In further studies in rabbits, Green et al. (1976) found that -9-THC dissolved in light or heavy mineral oil penetrates ocular tissues better than Tween 80 or sesame oil. A 0.1 percent solution of -9-THC produced an IOP reduction approximately equal to one marihuana cigarette. When the ophthalmic solution was applied to one eye, Green et al. found that the second eye had a lesser pressure reduction with a later onset, indicating systemic absorption of the drug.

Cooler and Gregg (1976) compared intravenous doses of 1.5 mg and 3 mg of -9-THC, 10 mg diazepam and a placebo in 10 normal volunteers. IOP was diminished 29 percent with the low and 37 percent with the high dosages of -9-THC. Diazepam lowered pressures 10 percent and the placebo 2 percent. These investigators also measured analgesia and noted no cutaneous or periosteal analgesic effects. The anxiety and dysphoria levels increased at both strengths of -9-THC, but not with diazepam or the placebo. Intravenous -9-THC appears to evoke anxiety much more often than when administered by the smoked or oral route.

Mechoulam et al. (1976) produced ocular hypertension in rabbits by means of -chymotrypsin injections into the eyeball. They tested a series of compounds and observed that 2 percent pilocarpine and 0.001 percent -9-THC were comparably potent while cannabidiol and cannabinol showed practically no effects.

As a matter of interest, the Food and Drug Administration (FDA), with the cooperation of NIDA and the Drug Enforcement Administration (DEA), has recently granted permission for a patient with glaucoma to be treated with marihuana cigarettes under an Investigational New Drug application from an ophthalmologist at Howard University. The subject was one of the patients in the previously cited study of Hepler et al. (1976), and was found to respond better to -9-THC than to the traditional anti-glaucoma medications.

Bronchodilation

Two lines of research, that of the Vachon group and the work of Tashkin and his collaborators, have clarified a number of questions about the effects of cannabis upon bronchial diameter. Vachon et al. (1973) observed the effects of a single administration of smoked marihuana on normal subjects and on asthmatic patients. They found that airway resistance decreased significantly in the normal group, permitting specific airway conductance and mean expiratory flow rates to increase. In the asthmatics bronchoconstriction was reversed for hours. From subsequent animal work, Vachon et al. (1976a) assume that the bronchodilation that follows -9-THC administration involves the adrenergic system. Recently, Vachon et al. (1976b, 1976c) used a microaerosolized -9-THC spray in 10 asthma. This aerosol was found to decrease airway resistance by an average of 16 percent at 90 minutes and increase flow rates without any significant tachycardia or high.

Tashkin et al. (1973) conducted a double blind study of 32 non-naive male subjects randomly assigned to groups smoking a placebo, using 1 percent -9-THC and 2 percent -9-THC. They found that both experimental dosages decreased airway resistance with a peak occurring 15 minutes after administration. Activity was still present after an hour. In a later study (1974), they examined dose-response curves with oral placebo, 10, 15 and 20 mg of -9-THC. Peak effects for the active drug were obtained at three hours with persisting effects for six hours.

Tashkin et al. (1975) also induced bronchospasm in asthmatics with either methacholine or exercise. Utilizing a single blind method, 10 mg of smoked -9-THC was compared with 1.25 mg of inhaled isoproterenol (Isuprel), both drugs having appropriate placebo controls. Bronchospasm was promptly relieved by both active drugs and not by their placebos. The isoproterenol had a quicker and higher peak effect, while -9-THC had a longer duration of action.

Tashkin et al. (1976b) also tried to clarify the mechanism of marihuana's bronchodilator action. In one set of experiments, 16 normal young males were either injected with atropine or smoked a cigarette containing 10 mg of -9-THC, and then received a methacholine challenge. In contrast to atropine, the -9-THC-induced increase in specific airway conductance was not blocked by methacholine.

In succeeding experiments, combinations of propanolol and -9-THC induced increases in specific airway conductance. This bronchodilator effect of cannabis may be independent of ß-adrenergic or antimuscarinic mechanisms.

In a recent article, Abboud and Sanders (1976) report on a double blind study involving six asthmatics and six control patients who were given oral -9-THC in 10 mg doses. They concluded that oral administration of -9-THC is unlikely to be of therapeutic value in asthma since its bronchodilator action is mild and inconstant. In addition, it is associated with significant CNS effects (mild depression and hangover). Moreover, one asthmatic patient in the study developed severe bronchoconstriction following the ingestion of -9-THC.

Tashkin et al. (1976b) and Olsen et al. (1975) have attempted to improve the delivery of -9-THC to the bronchioles by using an inhalation aerosol, since the use of marihuana cigarettes for this purpose is considered undesirable because of irritants, and possibly even carcinogens, in the smoke. Furthermore, the tachycardia end the psychic effects may not be desirable in asthmatics. A dose of 10 mg of -9-THC in a specially prepared aerosol produced substantial therapeutic levels of bronchodilation with lesser degrees of tachycardia and high than with a comparable oral amount. Unfortunately, the aerosol has a localized irritant effect that makes use in its current form undersirable.

Despite its bronchodilating effect, marihuana smoke is an irritant and, thus, interferes with other aspects of bronchial dynamics (Tashkin et al., 1976a). In addition, Huber et al. (1975) noted that alveolar macrophages harvested from rats by lavage, later incubated with Staphylococcus albus and graded amounts of marihuana smoke, caused a sustained dose-related depression of bactericidal activity. The reduction in bacterial macrophage activity was present in the gas phase and was water soluble. Further studies with purified -9-THC indicated that the impairment in alveolar macrophage function was not related to either the psychic or the bronchodilating components of marihuana.

Anticonvulsant

Most of the work investigating the anticonvulsant properties of cannabis has been preclinical. The effects of cannabinoids on animal seizures induced by pentylentetrazol (Metrazol), audiogenic or electrical stimulation have been recently examined. Consroe and his associates (Consroe et al., 1973, 1975b; Consroe & Man, 1973) found that -8- and -9-THC blocked all three types of seizures in a dose-related manner. These drugs were qualitatively comparable to diphenylhydantoin (Dilantin). Boggan et al. (1973) also confirmed the effect of -9-THC in mice with induced audiogenic seizures.

Dwivedi and Harbison (1975) found that -8- and -9-THC, marihuana extract and uridine protected against pentylentetrazol-induced convulsions in mice. None of these drugs protected against maximal electroshock-induced convulsions. The authors found that their anticonvulsant effects were not additive to diphenylhydantoin, but were additive to phenobarbital. Therefore, their mechanism of action may be similar to that of diphenylhydantoin but different from that of phenobarbital.

Sofia et al. (1976) determined that both -9-THC and diphenylhydantoin decrease polysynaptic transmission and post-tetanic potentiation. They concluded from their experiments on mice that there may be a clinical usefulness for a compound such as -9-THC which combines some degree of the anticonvulsant specificity of diphenylhydantoin with the general sedative effects of phenobarbital and chlordiazepoxide.

Rat hippocampal seizures precipitated by afferent electrical stimulation were studied by Feeney et al. (1973) to determine whether a series of cannabinoids would be effective. The cannabinoids were found to be more effective than diphenylhydantoin in diminishing the seizure discharges. Cannabidiol was the most potent, followed in order of effectiveness by cannabinol, -9-THC and -8-THC. In this study, the psychologically inactive cannabinoids outperformed the active ones.

Karler et al. (1973, 1974a, 1974b) demonstrated that tolerance developed to the antiseizure property in the maximal electroshock test. Their subjects were rats treated with -9-THC and mice treated with -9-THC, cannabidiol, diphenylhydantoin and pheno-barbital. In other electrical seizure models, tolerance was variable and specific for each model. Karler et al. considered it possible that cannabidiol, which has no psychotoxicity or cardiotoxicity, has the further advantage of being a better anticonvulsant than -9-THC. Turkanis and Karler (1975) investigated the post-tetanic potentiation of bullfrog paravertebral ganglia in vitro using 7-hydroxy-THC, 6 -7-dihydroxy-THC, -9-THC, cannabidiol, diphenylhydantoin and phenobarbital. Both hydroxy-THC metabolites and cannabidiol markedly depressed the post-tetanic potential at 30 to 90 minutes. Diphenylhydantoin depressed it moderately and -9-THC and phenobarbital had no effect. In this instance, the hydroxylated metabolites showed activity different from that of the parent compound.

Carlini et al. (1975) confirmed that cannabidiol may be the best cannabinoid anticonvulsant. Albino mice were administered transcorneal electroshocks and treated with either cannabidiol, cannabidiol-aldehyde acetate, 6-oxo-cannabidiol acetate, 6-hydroxycannabidiol triacetate or 9-hydroxy-cannabidiol triacetate. Cannabidiol and 6-oxo-cannabidiol acetate had the best anticonvulsant effect and therefore merit further study.

Johnson et al. (1975) determined the anticonvulsant activity of intravenous -9-THC in epileptic chickens by intermittent photic stimulation and pentylentetrazol. Cannabis reduced the severity and incidence of seizures produced by intermittent photic stimulation.

A reduction in frequency of inter-ictal, slow-wave, high voltage EEG; activity and an absence of spiking was also noted. -9-THC had no effect on the incidence of pentylentetrazol-induced seizures.

Ten Ham et al. (1975) gave 20 mg/kg of -9-THC for six days to gerbils with spontaneous epileptiform seizures. No effect was seen on the latency, duration or severity of the seizures. At a 50 mg/kg dose level, seizures were completely abolished after a single injection, but tolerance developed within six days. Severe toxicity occurred at the 50 mg/kg dosage level.

Wada et al. (1975) reported that -8-THC and -9-THC failed to affect the myoclonic response to photic stimulation in the Senegalese baboon. However, both drugs exerted dose-related antiepileptic effects upon established kindled convulsions provoked by electrical stimulation of the amygdala. The antiepileptic action of the two THC isomers appears to be caused by a suppression of propagation of the induced afterdischarge to distant cerebral structures, although high doses also suppress the afterdischarge at the site of stimulation. In previous investigations, Wada et al.

(1974) and Corcoran et al. (1973) had reported that -9-THC transiently suppresses the clinical and EEG seizure manifestations caused by subcortical stimulation in rats and cats.

Convulsant as well as anticonvulsant activity can be demonstrated with cannabinoids. The former is usually noted when toxic or high, chronic doses are used. However, Consroe et al. (1976) have bred a strain of New Zealand rabbit that is quite susceptible to -9-THC seizures. Doses of 0.1-0.8 mg/kg i.v. produced behavioral seizures regularly in these animals. In addition, spontaneously epileptic beagles were given varying doses of -9-THC, cannabidiol or a placebo for 20 days. Myoclonic jerks and generalized seizures were observed in those dogs receiving 3-5 mg/kg of -9-THC orally (Feeney et al. 1976).

Little work has been done in humans with cerebral dysrhythmias. The Davis and Ramsey (1949) study was a pilot effort that examined the effect of tetrahydrocannabinols in epileptic, hospitalized children who had been receiving diphenylhydantoin or mephenytoin (Mesantoin). Two children showed improvement on one cannabinoid, but transfer to a second cannabinoid gave mixed results. Perez-Reyes and Wingfield (1974), in a case report, mentioned that intravenously infused cannabidiol did not reduce, and may have increased, the abnormal EEG; activity of a 24-year-old man with centricephalic epilepsy. In this case, symmetrical spike and wave activity appeared only during light sleep. The 40 mg cannabidiol injection may have increased the dysrhythmia even though it produced a diminution in its intensity after awakening. Another case report (Consroe et al., 1975b) suggests that smoked marihuana may have a beneficial action in some types of human epilepsy. On the other hand, Keeler and Reifler (1967) suggest that marihuana may be detrimental in epileptics with grand mal convulsions. Feeney (1976) surveyed epileptics concerning illegal drug use. Practically none over 30 years of age reported illicit drug use, but 29 percent under 30 mentioned marihuana smoking. Only 4 percent had discussed the matter with their physicians. Most reported that it had no effect; one stated that it decreased epileptic seizures and another said that it caused his seizures.

The problems encountered with -9-THC (insolubility, variable oral absorption, psychotoxicity, tachycardia and the possibility of a convulsant capability) have resulted in the production of a series of synthesized benzopyrans. In particular, three analogues of dimethylheptylpyran (DMHP) were found to exhibit significant anticonvulsant activity against audiogenic, supramaximal electroshock and maximal pentylentetrazol-induced seizures in mice (Plotnikoff,1976). In rats, these compounds were found to be more active than diphenylhydantoin in the supramaximal electroshock test. One of them, SP-175, showed a different profile of anticonvulsant activity than DMHP or -9-THC. On the basis of five-day studies of diphenylhydantoin, phenobarbital, DMHP and SP-175 in mice, tolerance was not found to develop.

Retardation of Tumor Growth

Harris et al. (1976) have reported that mice innoculated with Lewis lung adenocarcinoma showed tumor size reductions ranging from 25-82 percent depending on the dose and duration of treatment with oral -8-THC, -9-THC and cannabinol. No reductions were found with cannabidiol. The effective cannabinoids increased survival time from one-quarter to one-third compared to a 50 percent increase with cyclophosphamide. Friend leukemia virus growth was inhibited by -9-THC, but L1210 murine leukemia was not. In vitro experiments confirmed the inhibition of neoplastic growth in mice, leading the authors to conclude that certain cannabinoids possess antineoplastic properties by virtue of their interference with RNA and DNA synthesis. In a later study (Harris, 1976), other tumor systems and other cannabinoids were tested. He found that cannabidiol seems to have a growth-enhancing, rather than reducing, effect on the Lewis lung tumor.

White et al. (1976), working with Lewis lung cell cultures exposed to -9-THC concluded that at non-toxic doses, the drug inhibits replication after thymidine uptake. This cytotoxicity may be relat e d t o -9-THC's extreme lipophilia, and, therefore, the results are related to effects on membrane function.

Antibacterial Activity

In an effort to replicate the work of Kabelik (1957) and Krejci (1958) mentioned earlier, van Klingeren and ten Ham (1976) tested the antibacterial activity of -9-THC and cannabidiol. Broth cultures of staphylococci and streptococci were innoculated with varying concentrations of -9-THC and cannabidiol. They found that both substances were bacteriostatic and bactericidal, but were ineffective against gram negative bacilli. When horse serum was incorporated, the antibacterial effect was greatly reduced, presumably due to protein binding. The utility of these cannabinoids as a topical antibacterial, as suggested by Krejci, seems to have been confirmed on an in vitro basis.

Those therapeutic studies that utilize the psychologic effects of marihuana follow.

Sedative-Hypnotic Action

Sofia and Knobloch (1973) demonstrated that pretreatment of laboratory animals with -9-THC reduces the dose of barbiturates needed for hypnosis and increases total sleep time. Freemon (1974) confirmed the observation of other investigators that -9-THC, like most hypnosedatives, reduces REM time. However, in contrast to other hypnotics, the abrupt withdrawal of -9-THC after six consecutive nights of usage failed to produce a REM rebound, although mild insomnia was observed.

Feinberg et al. (1976), using both marihuana extract and -9-THC, found that both drugs reduced REM activity and increased Stage IV sleep. Abrupt withdrawal led to considerably increased amounts of REM sleep and a transient decrease in Stage IV sleep. The difference in these findings from those of Freemon and others may be due to the large amounts of -9-THC given the subjects. Feinberg's subjects received from 70-210 mg per day.

In an attempt to exploit the well known relaxing and sedating effects of cannabis, two studies were performed by Neu et al. (1976). In the first study, nine subjects with sleep difficulties were given 10, 20 or 30 mg. of -9-THC or a placebo at weekly intervals using a double blind method. The drug, as compared to the placebo, significantly reduced sleep latency. Furthermore, sleep was less interrupted during the drug nights. Side effects were mild, but they increased with increasing dosage. The chief complaint was a hangover the next day. In the second study, the -9-THC doses were reduced to 5, 10 and 15 mg in order to avoid side effects. These were compared to a placebo and to 500 mg of chloral hydrate, a well-established hypnotic. Surprisingly, neither the chloral hydrate nor the -9-THC facilitated sleep induction or extended the duration of sleep as compared to the placebo. At the 15 mg dose level, a few complaints of hangover were noted. The authors suggested that difficulties in controlling the room temperature during the winter may have sufficiently interfered with sleep to negate any possible hypnotic effects of the active substances.

Tassinari et al. (1976) reported increases in total sleep time in eight volunteer subjects. Stage II sleep was increased while REM sleep was reduced. The dosages used were rather large (0.7- 1.0 mg/kg of -9-THC), however.

Analgesia

One of the earliest folk uses for cannabis was for pain relief. A series of preclinical investigations by Kaymakcalan et al. (1974) tended to confirm this analgesic effect. After having received intravenous administrations of 1 mg/kg -9-THC, dogs received electric stimulation through an implanted dental electrode. The cannabinoid produced a definite analgesic effect, as shown by a fourfold increase in pain thresholds. Tolerance to analgesia, sedation and ataxia occurred in eight days.

In another study, -9-THC produced pain reduction in mice and rats as measured by tail flick and writhing tests, and in rabbits receiving sciatic nerve stimulation. The analgesia produced with the doses used was equivalent to morphine analgesia -- in fact, in rats, a cross tolerance between -9-THC and morphine was found. An earlier study (Parker & Dubas, 1973) measured the effect of -9-THC on rats with electrodes implanted in aversive brain sites. A nondose related elevation of the pain threshold and an attenuation of the escape response were also recorded.

Sofia et al. (1975) tested the analgesic effectiveness of -9-THC, crude marihuana extract, cannabinol, cannabidiol, morphine and aspirin orally in mice using the acetic-induced writhing and the hot plate tests. They also exposed rats to the Randall-Selito paw pressure test. -9-THC and morphine were equipotent except in the paw pressure test in which morphine exceeded -9-THC in elevating the pain threshhold. The crude marihuana extract was as effective in all tests except in the acetic writhing test where it was three times more potent. Cannabinol resembled aspirin in that it was only efficacious in the writhing test.

A double blind Canadian study by Milstein et al. (1975) revealed a significant increase in pain tolerance among those who had smoked marihuana. Using a pressure algometer, the experimenter found that experienced subjects obtained greater analgesia than non-experienced subjects, although the increased pain tolerance was found only in the preferred hand. No effects on sensitivity to pain sensation were noted.

In another human study, Hill et al. (1974) recorded opposite results. Here, 26 subjects received blind, either marihuana smoke containing 12 mg of -9-THC from a spirometer or a marihuana placebo. They were then given electrical skin stimulation. The THC was found to decrease tolerance and heighten sensitivity to pain.

In an impressionistic report, Dunn and Davis (1974) questioned 10 paraplegics hospitalized in a V.A. hospital, all of whom had admitted using marihuana in the past. Four reported that it produced a decrease in phantom pain sensations, five mentioned a decrease in spasticity and five noted a decrease in headache pain and an increase in pleasant sensations.

Cancer patients in pain were studied by Noyes et al. (1975). Patients were given either -9-THC in 5, 10, 15 or 20 mg doses or a placebo. Pain reduction was greater at all -9-THC levels than in the placebo condition. Significant pain reduction was noted at the 15 and 20 mg THC levels. These researchers felt that the pain relief was not due to the sedative or euphoriant effects; and, therefore, attempted to compare the analgesic effect of 10 and 20 mg of -9-THC with 60 and 120 mg of codeine in a group of cancer patients with moderate pain. At the higher doses of both drugs, significant levels of analgesia were reported. The 20 mg dose of -9-THC produced marked sedation, and even the 10 mg dose was associated with considerable drowsiness. The sedation and mental effects of 20 mg of -9-THC preclude its therapeutic usefulness, but the investigators concluded that -9-THC has mild analgesic activity.

In a letter to the editor (Neiburg et al., 1976) in response to the Sallan et al. (1975) article on amelioration of nausea and vomiting by -9-THC in cancer chemotherapy patients, the writers tell of two patients with malignancies who had to stop smoking marihuana because of increased bone pain.

Wilson and May (1974) postulated 'that the analgesic activity of -8-and -9-THC resides primarily in their 11-hydroxy metabolites, the latter being three times more potent than the former. They based this assumption on the observation that 9-nor derivatives (which cannot be transformed into 11-hydroxy metabolites) lacked significant analgesic activity. These do exhibit dog ataxia and cardiovascular profiles nearly identical to -8- and -9-THC. This finding led to the preparation of 9-nor-9-ß-hydroxy-hexahydrocanna-binol which proved to be an analgesic in the mouse hot plate test nearly equal to morphine. Whether or not the analgesia occurs over an opiate receptor site is unresolved.

Harris (1976) was not able to confirm the analgesic effect of -9-THC using the standard analgesic test procedures. He did find the 9-nor-

9-ßhydroxyhexahydrocannabinol to be a potent antinocioceptive agent, confirming Wilson and May's work.

Pre-Anesthetic

A number of studies have examined the role that -9-THC can play as a pre-anesthetic agent, with mixed results. When it was given prior to inhalation anesthesia, the requirement for cyclopropane and halothane was decreased (Paton & Temple, 1973; Stoelting et al., 1973). Smith (1976) found that normal volunteers given 200 mcg/kg THC intravenously experienced marked sedation with minimal respiratory depression. Also salivation was diminished, bronchodilation occurred and cardiac output increased on the basis of the expected tachycardia. Although the author cautioned that some of the observed effects may have been due to the alcohol in which the -9-THC was dissolved, the amount of the drug given intravenously could easily have provided the manifestations recorded. Whether -9-THC has a potential usefulness in anesthesiology will depend on findings from additional studies.

Having searched for suitable pre-anesthetic combinations, Smith reported that 5 mg of -9-THC intravenously produced fear in a number of patients. In combination with an opioid it provided useful sedation, but with a marked decrease in carbon dioxide sensitivity. When combined with a barbiturate, the CNS depression was unpleasant and associated with some restlessness, but the response to carbon dioxide was unchanged. With diazepam, definite drowsiness and other depressive effects were notable, and the ventilatory response to carbon dioxide was decreased. The investigator suggested that the combination of marihuana with pre-anesthetic or anesthetic medications could lead to undesirable results.

Gregg and Small (1974) found two dosage levels of intravenous -9-THC ineffective in controlling anxiety in oral surgery patients. In fact, in low doses it elevated anxiety, sometimes to a marked degree. Intravenous diazepam out-performed the drug under investigation.

In an expansion of this study, Gregg et al. (1976b) found that the combination of presurgical stress and intravenous -9-THC produced dysphoria and a tendency to syncopal hypotension. No measurable effect on pain tolerance could be detected. The investigators concluded that surgical stress plus marihuana use immediately prior to the surgery might lead to psychophysiologic reactions.

Johnstone et al. (1975) also examined -9-THC in combination with other drugs. It was administered intravenously after subjects had been pretreated with oxymorphone (OXM) or pentobarbital (PBL). The sedative effects of OXM were increased by -9-THC, but the cannabinoid also increased respiratory depression. The combination of PBL and -9-THC did not cause respiratory depression but produced such intense anxiety and psychotomimetic reactions that four of the seven subjects receiving this combination were not given the full course of five doses. The investigators concluded that neither combination was a desirable anesthetic premeditation. They also expressed reservations about the value of -9-THC alone for such a purpose.

A number of reports in this area mention the cardio-accelerating effect of -9-THC as an undesirable feature of its activity. When it is combined with other drugs like atropine, and with the stress of pending surgery, syncopal hypotension can result. From a different perspective, Gregg and associates (1976a) mention that patients given general anesthesia within 72 hours of smoking marihuana sustained abnormal heart rate increases when compared with control non-smokers. They speculate that it could have resulted from an interaction between the stored cannabinoid metabolites and the various other elements of the surgical state that are conducive to tachycardia.

Antidepressant

Since marihuana tends to elevate mood, it follows that an evaluation of its antidepressant potential would be sought. Kotin et al. (1973) administered 0.3 mg/kg of -9-THC or a matching placebo twice daily to eight patients who required hospitalization for their affective disorder. The patients were all considered moderately or severely depressed. Treatment lasted a week, with placebos substituted for the active drug thereafter. No evidence of a significant affectual change could be demonstrated. In chronic depressive states, a longer duration of drug administration is sometimes needed before improvement is noted.

A group at the Medical College of Virginia (Regelson et al., 1976) performed a double blind study with cancer patients receiving chemotherapy. An initial starting dose of 0.1 mg/kg t.i.d. was used. The dosage was raised only if previous doses were welltolerated.

On a battery of personality tests and mood scales, the-9-THC acted as a mood elevator and tranquilizer producing significant improvement on two of three Zung depression scales.

Cognitive functioning was unimpaired and appetite enhancement and retardation of weight loss were noted from clinical records. The need for narcotics was decreased, and patients had the impression that some pain relief resulted.

Antinauseant, Antiemetic and Appetite Enhancer

The double blind Regelson study at the Medical College of Virginia is mentioned above in the section on antidepressant effects, but the researchers believed that the principal benefits seen in their cancer chemotherapy patients were the improvement of appetite and lack of the expected weight loss. Increased sociability and tranquilization were achieved by many patients according to the check lists used. Sedation, which could be desirable in this group of patients, was a frequent side effect. Nausea and vomiting were brought under control significantly more often by -9-THC than with the placebo.

Sallan et al. (1975) gave either oral -9-THC in 10 mg/sq. meter body surface or a placebo to 20 patients with each serving as his own control. An antiemetic effect was observed in 14 of the 20 drug courses, but not in the placebo courses. The antiemetic effect paralleled the subjective high. Studies comparing -9-THC with a standard antiemetic, prochlorperazine (Compazine), are underway at a few centers.

Treatment of Alcohol and Drug Dependence

Rosenberg (1976) has studied the response of a group of alcoholics and normal volunteers to marihuana cigarettes (0.4 gm/50 lb. body weight) and to alcohol (2 ml vodka/kg.). This investigator found that sober alcoholics tended to be less responsive to stresses (mental arithmetic and talking to a videocamera) and were more likely to withdraw from a stress situation than the normals.

Alcoholics became more angry and depressed after alcohol ingestion as measured by mood scales. Marihuana produced a more positive mood state and did not interfere with the arousal reaction, although it greatly increased heart rate and produced an acute paranoid or confusional state in 3 of the 27 subjects. This investigator also found that disulfiram (Antabuse) and marihuana could be given safely together in the treatment of alcoholism. The study is continuing, but the early findings indicate that marihuana may be a suitable therapeutic adjunct for some alcoholics as a reward to encourage them to take disulfiram.

Hine and colleagues (1975a) implanted morphine pellets in rats. -9-THC in 1, 2, 5 and 10 mg/kg doses were injected intraperitoneally 71 hours later. An hour afterwards, 4 mg/kg of naloxone (Narcan) was delivered into the same site. Attenuation of abstinence was achieved with a dose of 2 mg/kg and higher. Cannabidiol significantly potentiated the -9-THC effect on diarrhea and wet shakes.

In a letter, Carder (1975) criticized the paper by Hine on suppression of naloxone-precipitated morphine abstinence. He pointed out that only two of nine symptoms were reduced (wet shakes and defecations).

It was suggested that this could simply be a non-specific depressant effect . In reply, Hine et al. (1975b) stated that the decrease in wet shakes, diarrhea and bolus counts was dose related. The relative importance of one abstinence symptom over another is difficult to evaluate. Hine et al. retain the belief that a clinical trial of -9-THC in opiate detoxification is justified.

Bhargava (1976) has performed a similar study in mice. The naloxone precipitated jumping response was inhibited, and two other signs of morphine withdrawal (defecation and rearing behavior) were also suppressed by -9-THC. The author considers the jumping response to be a major sign of withdrawal.

The Synthetics

A long series of synthetic compounds has been developed over the past few years. They represent attempts to intensify certain desired activities of the tetrahydrocannabinols while avoiding the unwanted effects. Pars and Razdan (1976) have described. a series of nitrogen and sulfur substituted benzopyrans. Dren (1976) has studied the neuropharmacology of three nitrogen-containing heterocyclic benzopyrans and reported tranquilizing, analgesic, sedativehypnotic and intraocular pressure lowering activity. Plotnikoff et al. (1975) states that these nitrogen analogues have anticonvulsant properties in mice and rats. Nabilone, which has a ketone instead of a methyl on the 9 position of -9-THC, was investigated by Lemberger and Rowe (1976). It produced relaxation and sedative effects in humans. Little euphoria or tachycardia occurred, but in high doses postural hypotension developed. Tolerance to the euphoria and postural hypotension took place rapidly.

Mechanism of Therapeutic Action

The precise mechanism by which cannabis exerts its pharmacologic effects remains unknown. Burstein and Raz (1972) and Burstein et al. (1973) have gathered a considerable amount of indirect evidence that some of the actions are mediated via a prostaglandin-cyclic AMP system. He found that -9-THC reduced prostaglandin formation by inhibiting prostaglandin synthetase. Other cannabinoids have this effect as does olivetol from which -9-THC is synthesized. PGE2 and PGE1 are two of the prostaglandins affected. Prostaglandin inhibition could account for the intraocular pressure reducing and the bronchodilating actions.

The influence of cannabinoids upon neurotransmitters has been examined, but the results are inconsistent. Banerjee et al. (1975) have shown in vitro that -8- and -9-THC and their hydroxylated metabolites inhibit the uptake of norepinephrine and serotonin in hypothalamic synaptosome preparations and of dopamine in the corpus striatum. Gamma-aminobutyric acid uptake in cerebral cortical preparations is also inhibited. The latter may explain the anticonvulsant properties of some of the cannabinoids. Drew and Miller (1974) believe that cholinergic dominance best explains the mental effects. The adrenergic activity of cannabis mentioned earlier (Green & Kim, 1976) is not inconsistent with the prostaglandincyclic

AMP hypothesis; rather, it may be an antecedent reaction to the release of adrenergic amines. Selective monoamine oxidase inhibitory activity is also a possible feature of some activity of the cannabinoids (Schurr and Livne, 1975).

CONCLUSION

The further study of the cannabinoids for various therapeutic applications seems worthwhile. A large number of synthetic cannabinoids have begun to appear which do not have some of the disadvantages intrinsic in the naturally occurring ones. Therapeutic efficacy could be enhanced by certain molecular manipulations.

Thus, it is likely that if any cannabinoid ever achieves clinical acceptance, it will be a synthetic.

The cannabinoid configuration would be important to human therapeutics because: 1) there is a wide safety margin between effective and lethal doses, and 2) in certain instances, the mechanism of action appears to differ from the standard medications now employed.

It should be noted that successful clinical trials of cannabis or its constituents do not provide sufficient justification for removal of the drug from Schedule I (no medical usefulness, high abuse potential) to a less restricted scheduled. Only when the substance has gone through the entire investigational process of testing, and the FDA has approved its New Drug Application, would its rescheduling be considered by the regulatory agencies.

Sidney Cohen, M.D., D.Sc.

University of California

at Los Angeles

REFERENCES

Therapeutic Aspects

Abboud, R.T. and Sanders, H.D. Effect of oral administration of -9-tetrahydrocannabinol on airway mechanics in normal and asthmatic subjects. Chest, 70:480-485 (1976).

Agurell, S., Gustafsson, B., Holmstedt, B., Leander, K., Lindgren, J.-E., Nilsson, I., Sandberg, F. and Asberg, M. Quantitation of 1-tetrahydrocannabinol in plasma from cannabis smokers. Journal of Pharmacy and Pharmacology, 25:554-558 (1973).

Banerjee, S.P., Snyder, S.H. and Mechoulam, R. Cannabinoids: Influence on neurotransmitter uptake in rat brain synaptosomes. Journal of Pharmacology and Experimental Therapeutics, 194:74-81 (1975).

Bhargava, H.N. Inhibition of naloxone-induced withdrawal in morphine dependent mice by 1-trans- -9-tetrahydrocannabinol. European Journal of Pharmacology, 38:259-262 (1976). Birch, E.A. The use of Indian hemp in the treatment of chronic chloral and chronic opium poisoning. Lancet, 1:625 (1889).

Boggan, W.O., Steele, R.A. and Freedman, D.X. -9-tetrahydrocannabinol effect on audiogenic seizure susceptibility. Psychopharmacologia, 29:101-106 (1973).

Burstein, S., Levin, E. and Varanelli, C. Prostaglandins and cannabis: Inhibition of biosynthesis by the naturally occurring cannabinoids. Biochemical Pharmacology, 22:2905-2910 (1973).

Burstein, S. and Raz, A. Inhibition of Prostaglandin E2 biosynthesis by -9-THC. Prostaglandins, 2:369-374 (1972).

Carder, B. Blockade of morphine abstinence by -9-tetrahydrocannabinol. Science, 190:590 (1975).

Carlini, E.A., Mechoulam, R. and Lander, N. Anticonvulsant activity of four oxygenated cannabidiol derivatives. Research Communications in Chemical Pathology and Pharmacology, 12(1):1-15 (1975).

Cohen, S. The sex-pot controversy. Drug Abuse and Alcoholism Newsletter, 6(4):1-4 (1975).

Cohen, S. and Stillman, R.C. (eds.) The Therapeutic Potential of Marihuana. New York: Plenum, 1976.

Consroe, P.F., Jones, B.C. and Chin, L. -9-tetrahydrocannabinol, EEG and behavior: The importance of adaptation to the testing milieu. Pharmacology, Biochemistry and Behavior, 3:173-177 (1975a).

Consroe, P.F., Jones, B.C., Laird, H. and Reinking, J. Anticonvulsant-convulsant effects of -9-tetrahydrocannabinol. In Cohen, S. and Stillman, R.C. (eds.), The Therapeutic Potential of Marihuana. New York: Plenum, 1976, pp. 343-362.

Consroe, P.F. and Man, D.P. Effects of -8- and -9-tetrahydrocannabinol on experimentally induced seizures. Life Sciences, 13:429-439 (1973).

Consroe, P.F., Man, D.P., Chin, L. and Picchioni, A.L. Reduction of audiogenic seizures by -8- and -9-tetrahydrocannabinol. Journal of Pharmacy and Pharmacology, 25:764-765 (1973).

Consroe, P.F., Wood, G.C. and Buchsbaum, H. Anticonvulsant nature of marihuana smoking. Journal of the American Medical Association, 234:306-307 (1975b).

Cooler, P. and Gregg, J.M. The effect of -9-tetrahydrocannabinol on intraocular pressure in humans. In Cohen, S. and Stillman, R.C. (eds.), The Therapeutic Potential of Marihuana. New York: Plenum, 1976, pp. 77-88.

Corcoran, M.E., McCaughran, J.A. and Wada, J.A. Acute antiepileptic effects of -9-tetrahydrocannabinol in rats with kindled seizures. Experimental Neurology, 40:471-483 (1973).

Davis, J.P. and Ramsey, H.H. Antiepileptic action of marihuana active substances. Federation Proceedings, 8:284-285 (1949).

Dren, A.T. Preclinical neuropharmacology of three nitrogen-containing heterocyclic benzopyrans derived from the cannabinoid nucleus. In Cohen, S. and Stillman, R.C. (eds.), The Therapeutic Potential of Marihuana. New York: Plenum, 1976, pp.

Drew, W.G. and Miller, L.L. Cannabis: Neural mechanisms and behavior, a theoretical review. Pharmacology, 11:12-13 (1974).

Dunn, D. and Davis, R. The perceived effects of marihuana in spinal cord injuries. Paraplegia, 12:175 (1974).

Dwivedi, C. and Harbison, R.D. Anticonvulsant activities of -8-and -9-tetrahydrocannabinol and uridine. Toxicology and Applied Pharmacology, 31:452-458 (1975).

Emboden, W.A.V. Ritual use of cannabis sativa L.: A historical ethnographic survey. In Furst, P. (ed.), Flesh of the Gods.New York: Praeger, 1972.

Feeney, D.M. Marihuana use among epileptics. Journal of the American Medical Association, 235:1105 (1976).

Feeney, D.M., Spiker, M. and Weiss, G.K. Marihuana and epilepsy: Activation of symptoms by -9-THC. In Cohen, S. and Stillman, R.C. (eds.), The Therapeutic Potential of Marihuana. New York: Plenum, 1976, pp. 343-362.

Feeney, D.M., Wagner, H.R., McNamara, M.C. and Weiss, G. Effects of tetrahydrocannabinol on hippocampal evoked after discharges in cats. Experimental Neurology, 41:357-365 (1973).

Feinberg, I., Jones, R., Walker, J., Cavness, C. and Floyd, T.

Effects of marihuana extract and tetrahydrocannabinol on electroencephalographic sleep patterns. Clinical Pharmacology and Therapeutics, 19:782-794 (1976).

Flom, M.C., Adams, A.J. and Jones, R.T. Marihuana smoking and reduced pressure in human eyes: Drug action or epiphenomenon? Investigative Ophthalmology, 14:52-55 (1975).

Freemon, F.R. The effect of -9-tetrahydrocannabinol on sleep. Psychopharmacologia, 35:39-44 (1974).

Green, K. Marihuana and the eye. Investigative Ophthalmology, 14:261-263 (1975).

Green, K. and Kim, K. Interaction of adrenergic blocking agents with prostaglandin E2 and tetrahydrocannabinol in the eye. Experimental Eye Research, 15:499-507 (1973).

Green, K. and Kim, K. Interaction of adrenergic antagonists with prostaglandin E2 and tetrahydrocannabinol in the eye. Investigative Ophthalmology, 15:102-111 (1976).

Green, K., Kim, K. and Bowman, K. Ocular effects of -9-tetrahydrocannabinol. In Cohen, S. and Stillman, R.C. (eds.), The Therapeutic Potential of Marihuana. New York: Plenum, 1976, pp. 49-62.

Green, K. and Podos, S.M. Antagonism of arachidonic acid-induced ocular effects by -9-tetrahydrocannabinol. Investigative Ophthalmology, 13:422-429 (1974).

Gregg, J.M., Campbell, R.L., Levin, K.J., Ghia, J. and Elliott, R.A. Cardiovascular effects of cannabinol during oral surgery. Anesthesia and Analgesia, 55:203-213 (1976a).

Gregg, J.M. and Small, E.W. The control of anxiety in oral surgery patients with -9-THC and diazepam. NIH Record, 26:8 (1974).

Gregg, J.M., Small, E.W., Moore, R., Raft, D. and Toomey, T.C. Emotional response to intravenous -9-tetrahydrocannabinol during oral surgery. Journal of Oral Surgery, 34:301-313 (1976b).

Grinspoon, L. Marihuana Reconsidered. Cambridge: Harvard University Press, 1971. Harris, L.S. Analgesic and antitumor potential of the cannabinoids. In Cohen, S. and Stillman, R.C. (eds), The Therapeutic Potential of Marihuana. New York: Plenum, 1976, pp. 299-312.

Harris, L.S., Munson, A.E. and Carchman, R.A. Anti-tumor properties of cannabinoids. In Braude, M.C. and Szara, S. (eds.), Pharmacology of Marihuana. New York: Raven Press, 1976, pp.749-762.

Hepler, R.S. and Frank, I.M. Marihuana smoking and intraocular pressure. Journal of the American Medical Association, 217:1392 (1971).

Hepler, R.S., Frank, I.M., and Petrus, R. Ocular effects of marihuana smoking. In Braude, M.C. and Szara, S. (eds.), Pharmacology of Marihuana. New York: Raven Press, 1976, pp. 815-824.

Hill, S.Y., Schwin, R., Goodwin, D.W. and Powell, B.J. Marihuana and pain. Journal of Pharmacology and Experimental Therapeutics, 188:415-418 (1974).

Hine, B., Friedman, E., Torrelio, M. and Gershon, S. Morphinedependent rats: Blockade of precipitated abstinence by tetrahydrocannabinol. Science, 187:443-446 (1975a).

Hine, B., Friedman, E., Torrelio, M. and Gershon, S. Blockade of precipitated abstinence by tetrahydrocannabinol. Science, 190:591 (1975b).

Hubacek, J. Study of the effect of cannabis indica in oto-rhinolaryngology. Acta Univ. Olomuc. Fac. Med., 6:83-86 (1955).

Huber, G.L., Simmons, G.A., McCarthy, C.R., Cutting, M.B.,

Laguarda, R. and Pereira, W. Depressant effects of marihuana smoke on antibacterial activity of pulmonary alveolar macrophages. Chest, 68:769-773 (1975).

Johnson, D.D., McNeil, J.R., Crawford, R.D. and Wilcox, W.C. Epileptiform seizures in domestic fowl: Anticonvulsant activity of -9-tetrahydrocannabinol. Canadian Journal of Physiology and Pharmacology, 53:1007-1013 (1975).

Johnstone, R.E., Lief, P.L., Kulp, R.A. and Smith, T.C. Combination of -9-tetrahydrocannabinol with oxymorphone or phenobarbital: Effects on ventilatory control and cardiovascular dynamics. Anesthesiology, 42:674-684 (1975).

Kabelik, J.O. Hemp - its history - traditional and popular application. Acta Univ. Olomuc Fac. Med., 6:31-41 (1955).

Kabelik, J.O. Hanf (cannabis sativa) - antibiotishes heilmittel.1. Mitteilung: hanf in der alt - und volksmedizin. Die Pharmazie, 12:439 (1957).

Kabelik, J.O., Krejci, Z. and Santavy, F. Hemp as a medicament. Bulletin on Narcotics, 12:5-22 (1960).

Karler, R., Cely, W. and Turkanis, S.A. The anticonvulsant activity of cannabidiol and cannabinol. Life Sciences, 13:1527-1531 (1973).

Karler, R., Cely, W. and Turkanis, S.A. Anticonvulsant properties of -9-tetrahydrocannabinol and other cannabinoids. Life Sciences, 15:931-947 (1974a).

Karler, R., Cely, W. and Turkanis, S.A. A study of the development of tolerance to an anticonvulsant effect of -9-tetrahydrocannabinol and cannabidiol. Research Communications in Chemical Pathology and Pharmacology, 9:23-39 (1974b).

Kaymakcalan, S., Turker, R.K. and Turker, M.N. Analgesic effect of-9-tetrahydrocannabinol and development of tolerance to this effect in the dog. Psychopharmacologia, 35:123-128 (1974).

Keeler, M.H. and Reifler, C.F. Grand mal convulsions subsequent to marihuana use. Diseases of the Nervous System, 28:474-475 (1967).

Kolodny, R.C., Lessin, P., Toro, G., Masters, W.H. and Cohen, S. Depression of plasma testosterone with acute marihuana administration. In Braude, M.C. and Szara, S. (eds.), Pharmacology of Marihuana. New York: Raven Press, 1976, pp. 217-

Kotin, J., Post, R.M. and Goodwin, F.K. -9-tetrahydrocannabinol in depressed patients. Archives of General Psychiatry, 28:345-348 (1973).

Krejci, Z. The antibiotic effect of cannabis indica. Dissertation(Masaryk University, Brno), (1950).

Krejci, Z. The antibacterial effect of cannabis indica. Lekarske Listy, 1(20):500-503 (1952).

Krejci, Z. The antibacterial effect of cannabis indica. Acta Univ. Olomuc. Fac. Med., 6:43-57 (1955).

Krejci, Z. Hanf (cannabis sativa) - antibiotishes heilmittel. 2.

Mitteilung: Methodik und ergebnisse der bakteriologishen untersuchung und vorlaufige klinishe erfahrugen. Die Pharmazie, 13:155-156 (1958).

Krejci, Z. Antibacterial substances of cannabis used in the prevention and therapy of infections. Dissertation, 259 (1961a).

Krejci, Z. To the problem of substances with antibacterial and hashish effect in hemp. Casopis Lekaru Ceskych, 43:1351-1354 (1961b).

Krejci, Z. and Heczko, P. On the treatment of the papilla rhagades in suckling puerperial mothers and on the prevention of mastitis caused by staphylococci. Acta Univ. Olomuc. Fac. Med., 14:277-282 (1958).

Krejci, Z., Horok, M. and Santavy, F.I. Hanf (cannabis sativa) -antibiotishes heilmittel. 3. Mitteilung: Isolierung und

Konstitution zweier aus cannabis sativa gewonnener sauren. Die Pharmazie, 14:349-355 (1959).

Krejci, Z. and Vybiral, L. Thin layer (aluminum oxide) chromatographic isolation of biological active substances from cannabis sativa L. and the biological retention of antibacterially active substances. Scr. Med. Brno., 35:71-72 (1962).

Lemberger, L. and Rowe, H. Clinical pharmacology of nabilone, a cannabinol derivative. Clinical Pharmacology and Therapeutics, 18:720-726 (1976).

Mattison, J.B. Cannabis indica as an anodyne and hypnotic. St. Louis Medical and Surgical Journal, 61:265-271 (1891).

Mechoulam, R. and Gaoni, Y. A total synthesis of dl- -1-tetrahydrocannabinol, the active constituent in hashish. Journal of the American Chemical Society, 87:3273-3275 (1965).

Mechoulam, R., Lander, N., Dikstein, S., Carlini, E. and Blumenthal, M. On the therapeutic possibilities of some cannabinoids. In Cohen, S. and Stillman, R.C. (eds.), The Therapeutic Potential of Marihuana. New York: Plenum, 1976, pp. 35-48.

Mechoulam, R., Shani, A., Edery, H. and Grunfeld, Y. Chemical basis of hashish activity. Science, 169:611-612 (1970).

Milstein, S.L., MacCannell, K., Karr, G. and Clark, S. Marihuana produced changes in pain tolerance: Experienced and nonexperienced subjects. International Pharmacopsychiatry (Basel), 10:177-182 (1975).

M'Meens, R.R. Report on the Committee on cannabis indica. Transactions of the Fifteenth Annual Meeting of the Ohio State Medical Society, 15:75-100 (1860).

Moreau de Tours, J.J. Psychotic depression with stupor tendency to dementia: Treatment with an extract of cannabis indica. Lancette Hospital Gazette, 30:391 (1857).

Navratil, J. Effectiveness of cannabis indica on chronic otitis media. Acta Univ. Olomuc. Fac. Med., 6:87-89 (1955).

Neiburg, H.A., Margolin, F. and Seligman, B.R. Tetrahydrocannabinol and Chemotherapy. New England Journal of Medicine, 294: 168 (1976).

Neu, C., DiMascio, A., and Zwilling, G. Hypnotic properties of THC: Experimental comparison of THC with chloral hydrate and placebo. In Cohen, S. and Stillman, R.C. (eds.), The Therapeutic Potential of Marihuana. New York: Plenum, 1976, pp.153-160.

Noyes, R., Brunk, S.F., Baram, D.A. and Canter, A. Analgesic effect of -9-tetrahydrocannabinol. The Journal of Clinical Pharmacology, 15:139-143 (1975).

Olsen, J.L., Lodge, J.W., Shapiro, B.J. and Tashkin, D.P. An inhalation aerosol of -9-tetrahydrocannabinol. Journal of Pharmacy and Pharmacology, 28:86 (1975).

O'Shaughnessy, W.B. On the preparation of the Indian hemp or Gunjah (cannabis indica). Transactions of the Medical and Physical Society of Bombay, 8:421-461 (1842).

Parker, C.S. and Wrigley, F. Synthetic cannabis preparations in psychiatry: Synhexyl. Journal of Mental Science, 96:276-279 (1950).

Parker, J.M. and Dubas, T.C. Automatic determination of the pain threshold to electroshock and the effects of -9-THC. International Journal of Clinical Pharmacology, Therapy and Toxicology, 7(1):75-81 (1973).

Pars, H. and Razdan, R. Heterocyclic analogues of the cannabinoids. In Cohen, S. and Stillman, R.C. (eds.), The Therapeutic Potential of Marihuana. New York: Plenum, 1976, pp. 419-488.

Paton, W.D.M. and Temple, D.M. Effects of chronic and acute cannabis treatment upon thiopentane anesthesia in rabbits.

Proceedings of the British Pharmacological Society (1973).

Perez-Reyes, M. and Wingfield, M. Cannabidiol and electroencephalographic epileptic activity. Journal of the American Medical Association, 230:1635 (1974).

Plotnikoff, N.P. New benzopyrans: Anticonvulsant activities. In Cohen, S. and Stillman, R.C. (eds.), The Therapeutic Potential of Marihuana. New York: Plenum, 1976, pp. 475-494.

Plotnikoff, N.P., Zaugg, H.E., Petersen, A.C., Arendsen, D.L. and Anderson, R.F. New benzopyrans: Anticonvulsant activities. Life Sciences, 17:97-104 (1975).

Procek, J. Preliminary study on the local effect of cannabis indica: A remedy for specific fistulas. Acta Univ. Olomuc. Fac. Med., 6:91-92 (1955).

Purnell, W.D. and Gregg, J.M. -9-tetrahydrocannabinol, euphoria and intraocular pressure in man. Annals of Ophthalmology, 7:921-923 (1975).

Quimby, M.W., Doorenbos, N.J., Turner, C.E. and Masoud, A. Mississippi grown marihuana cannabis sativa: Cultivation and observed morphological variations. Economic Botany, 27:117-127 (1973).

Regelson, W., Butler, J.R., Schultz, J., Kirk, T., Peck, L., Green, M.L. and Zakis, O. -9-tetrahydrocannabinol as an effective antidepressant and appetite stimulating agent in advanced cancer patients. In Braude, M.C. and Szara, S. (eds.),

Pharmacology of Marihuana. New York: Raven Press, 1976, pp.763-776.

Report of the Indian Hemp Drugs Commission, 1893-1894. Reprinted Silver Spring, MD: Thomas Jefferson Press, 1969.

Reynolds, J.R. Therapeutic uses and toxic effects of cannabis indica. Lancet, 1:637-638 (1890).

Rosenberg, C.M. The use of marihuana in the treatment of alcoholism. In Cohen, S. and Stillman, R.C. (eds.), The Therapeutic Potential of Marihuana. New York: Plenum, 1976, pp.173-182.

Rubin, V. Cross-cultural perspectives on therapeutic uses of cannabis. In Cohen, S. and Stillmen, R.C. (eds.), The Therapeutic Potential of Marihuana. New York: Plenum, 1976, pp. 1-18.

Rubin, V. and Comitas, L. Ganja in Jamaica. The Hague: Mouton, 1975.

Sallan, S.E., Zinberg, N.E. and Frei, E. Antiemetic effect of -9-tetrahydrocannabinol in patients receiving cancer chemotherapy. New England Journal of Medicine, 293(16):795-797 (1975).

Schurr, A. and Livne, A. Differential inhibition of mitochondrial monoamine oxidase from brain by hashish components. Israeli Journal of Medical Sciences, 11:1188 (1975).

Shapiro, D. The ocular manifestations of the cannabinols. Ophthalmologica, 168:366-369 (1974).

Simek, J. Application of the cannabis indica extract in preserving stomatology. Acta Univ. Olcmuc. Fac. Med., 6:79-82 (1955).

Sirek, J. Importance of hempseeds in the tuburculosis therapy. Acta Univ. Olomuc Fac. Med., 6:93-108 (1955).

Smith, T.C. Respiratory and cardiovascular effects of -9-tetrahydrocannabinol alone and in combination with oxymorphone, pentobarbital and diazepma. In Cohen, S. and Stillman, R.C. (eds.), The Therapeutic Potential of Marihuana. New York: Plenum, 1976, pp. 123-132.

Sofia, R.D. and Knobloch, L.C. The interaction of -9-tetrahydrocannabinol pretreatment with various sedative-hypnotic drugs. Psychopharmacologia, 30:185-194 (1973).

Sofia, R., Soloman, T. and Perry, H. Anticonvulsant activity of -9-THC compared with three other drugs. European Journal of Pharmacology, 35:7-10 (1976).

Sofia, R.D., Vassar, H.B. and Knobloch, L.C. Comparative analgesic activity of various naturally occurring cannabinoids in mice and rats. Psychopharmacologia, 40:285-295 (1975).

Soldan, J. Therapeutic results in stomatology after application of substances obtained from cannabis indica. Acta Univ. Olomuc. Fac. Med., 6:73-78 (1955).

Stoelting, R.K., Martz, R.C., Gartner, J., Creasser, C., Brown, D.J. and Forney, R.B. Effects of -9-tetrahydrocannabinol on halothane MAC in dogs. Anesthesiology, 38:521-523 (1973).

Tashkin, D.P., Shapiro, B. J. and Frank, I.M. Acute pulmonary physiologic effects of smoked marihuana and oral -9-tetrahydrocannabinol.

New England Journal of Medicine, 289:336-341 (1973).

Tashkin, D.P., Shapiro, B.J. and Frank, I.M. Acute effects of smoked marihuana and oral -9-tetrahydrocannabinol: Mechanisms of increased specific airway conductance in asthmatic subjects. American Review of Respiratory Disease, 109:420-428 (1974).

Tashkin, D.P., Shapiro, B. J., Lee, Y.E. and Harper, C.E. Effects of smoked marijuana in experimentally induced asthma. American Review of Respiratory Disease, 112:377-387 (1975).

Tashkin, D.P., Shapiro, B.J., Lee, Y.E. and Harper, C.E. Subacute effects of heavy marihuana smoking on pulmonary function in healthy men. New England Journal of Medicine, 294:125-129 (1976a).

Tashkin, D.P., Shapiro, B.J., Reiss, S., Olsen, J. and Lodge, J. Bronchial effects of aerosolized -9-tetrahydrocannabinol. In Cohen, S. and Stillman, R.C. (eds.), The Therapeutic Potential of Marihuana. New York: Plenum, 1976b, pp. 97-110.

Tassinari, C.A., Ambrosetto, G., Peraita-Adrados, M.R. and Gastaut, H. The neuropsychiatric syndrome of -9-tetrahydrocannabinol and cannabis intoxication in naive subjects: A clinical and polygraphic study during wakefulness and sleep. In Braude, M.C. and Szara, S. (eds.), Pharmacology of Marihuana. New York: Raven Press, 1976, pp. 357-375.

Ten Ham, M., Loskota, W.J. and Lomax, P. Acute and chronic effects of -9-tetrahydrocannabinol on seizures in the gerbil. European Journal of Pharmacology, 31:148-152. (1975).

Thompson, L.J. and Proctor, R.C. Pyrahexyl in the treatment of alcoholic and drug withdrawal conditions. North Carolina Medical Journal, 14:520-523 (1967).

Turkanis, S. and Karler, P. Influence of anticonvulsant cannabinoids in posttetanic potentiation at isolated bullfrog ganglia. Life Sciences, 17:569-578 (1975).

Vachon, L., FitzGerald, M.X., Solliday, N.H., Gould, I.A. and Gaensler, E.A. Single dose effect of marihuana smoke. New England Journal of Medicine, 288:985-989 (1973).

Vachon, L., Malthe, A. and Weissman, B. Effect of -9-THC on the catecholamine content of the guinea pig lung. Research Communications in Chemical Pathology and Pharmacology, 13:345-348 (1976a).

Vachon, L., Robins, A. and Gaensler, E. Airways response to aerosolized -9-tetrahydrocannabinol: Preliminary report. In Cohen, S. and Stillman, R.C. (eds.), The Therapeutic Potential of Marihuana. New York: Plenum, 1976b, pp. 111-122.

Vachon, L., Robins, A. and Gaensler, E.A. Airways response to micro-aerosolized -8-tetrahydrocannabinol. Chest, 70:444 (1976c).

Van Klingeren, B. and Ten Ham, M. Antibacterial activity of -9-tetrahydrocannabinol and cannabidiol. Antonie van Leeuwenhoek, 42:9-11 (1976).

Wada, J.A., Asawa, T. and Corcoran, M.E. Effects of tetrahydrocannabinols on kindled amygdaloid seizures and photogenic seizures in Senegalese baboons, Papio papio. Epilepsia, 16:439-448 (1975).

Wada, J.A., Sato, M., Green, J. and Troupin, A. Anticonvulsive and prophylactic potency of antiepileptic agents assessed by amygdaloid kindling in cats. Epilepsia, 15:276 (1974).

White, A., Munson, J., Munson, A. and Carchman, R. Effects of -9-tetrahydrocannabinol in Lewis lung adenocarcinoma cells in tissue culture. Journal of the National Cancer Institute, 56:655-658 (1976).

Wilson, R.S. and May, E.L. 9-nor- -8-tetrahydrocannabinol: A cannabinoid of metabolic interest. Journal of Medical Chemistry, 17:475-476 (1974). 17:475-476 (1974).

CONCLUSION
An Analysis taken from: **The Real Reason Cannabis Has Not Been Rescheduled: A Cure For Cancer Delayed?**

If substances in Cannabis can cure cancer, and research has been delayed by current law, the United States Government is partially culpable in 390,000 deaths each year. Furthermore, there are several deadly conditions Cannabis could possibly treat, according to literature released from the National Institute of Drug Abuse in 1977. As quoted in the second section of this book, the publication "Marihuana Research Findings: 1976" reveals that these conditions can be treated by Cannabis:

Bronchodilation
Anticonvulsant
Analgesia
Antidepressant
Treatment of Alcohol and Drug Dependence

The 1977 report also affirms that Cannabis has anti-tumor activity, an admission of anti-cancer effects. It also acknowledges marijuana as an anti-nausea medication, which would also save lives. The U.S. Government however, has developed a synthetic cannabinoid, Marinol, to be used for nausea. The government had to petition the United Nations to reschedule this substance. So, they have helped save some lives by this action.

It is possible the some of the lives lost in the five categories listed above could have been saved. Failure to invest in the development of new medications from Cannabis to treat these conditions possibly has resulted in the deaths of thousands of men, women, and children. Let's consider the deaths caused by each of these conditions:

1. Bronchodilation
This means opening up the air passages, and lungs, i.e. it can help with asthma. Two years before NIDA's report, a study was completed that concluded that marijuana could treat asthma:

Effects of smoked marijuana in experimentally induced asthma.
American Review of Respiratory Disease
Tashkin DP, Shapiro BJ, Lee YE, Harper CE
September 1975.

Abstract:
"After experimental induction of acute bronchospasm in 8 subjects with clinically stable bronchial asthma, effects of 500 mg of smoked marijuana (2.0 per cent delta9-tetrahydrocannabinol) on specific airway conductance and thoracic gas volume were compared with those of 500 mg of smoked placebo marijuana (0.0 per cent delta9-tetrahydrocannabinol), 0.25 ml of aerosolized saline, and 0.25 ml of aerosolized isoproterenol (1,250 mug). Bronchospasm was induced on 4 separate occasions, by inhalation of methacholine and, on four other occasions, by exercise on a bicycle ergometer or treadmill. Methacholine and exercise caused average decreases in specific airway conductance of 40 to 55 per cent and 30 to 39 per cent, respectively, and average increases in thoracic gas volume of 35 to 43 per cent and 25 to 35 per cent, respectively. After methacholine-induced bronchospasm, placebo marijuana and saline inhalation produced minimal changes in specific airway conductance and thoracic gas volume, whereas 2.0 per cent marijuana and isoproterenol each caused a prompt correction of the bronchospasm and associated hyperinflation. After exercise-induced bronchospasm, placebo marijuana and saline were followed by gradual recovery during 30 to 60 min, whereas 2.0 per cent marijuana and isoproterenol caused an immediate reversal of exercise-induced asthma and hyperinflation 36 ."

Another study reported similar results. In a 1973 article published in the New England Journal of Medicine, titled "Single-Dose Effect of Marihuana Smoke—Bronchial Dynamics and Respiratory-Center Sensitivity in Normal Subjects" we read:

> "Normal volunteers with previous marihuana smoking experience inhaled the total smoke from 3.23 mg per kilogram of marihuana, using a bag-in-box technic. Randomly, nine received marihuana containing a high (2.6 per cent), and eight a low (1.0 per cent) concentration of delta-9 tetrahydrocannabinol. Physiologic variables were monitored before and for 20 minutes after smoking. In the high-dose group the heart rate increased 28 per cent. Concomitantly, airway resistance, measured in a body plethysmograph, fell 38 per cent; the functional residual capacity remained unchanged (± 50 ml) throughout, and specific airway conductance increased 44 per cent. Flow-volume loops showed a 45 per cent increase in flow rate at 25 per cent of vital capacity. The low-dose group showed no increase in heart rate but significant, if lesser changes, in airways

dynamics. Carbon dioxide sensitivity, measured by rebreathing remained unchanged in both groups. Marihuana smoke, unlike cigarette smoke, causes bronchodilatation rather than bronchoconstriction and, unlike opiates, does not cause central respiratory depression." (New England Journal of Medicine 288:985–989, 1973)

These subjects were given a very low dose of marijuana, which means they had to smoke more to achieve the same effect of a few puffs of higher potency Cannabis. Nevertheless, the ability to treat asthma with Cannabis was noted in 1974, and reported to Congress in 1977. Yet, Marijuana continued to be placed in the most restrictive Schedule, which made further studies into this issue rare.

The inability to treat asthma effectively results in 250,000 deaths each year. If Cannabis can treat asthma, the United States government partially to blame for these deaths. They had evidence, and did nothing about it. Furthermore, as many as 80 percent of these deaths might be caused by the asthma medications:

"Three common asthma inhalers containing the drugs salmeterol or formoterol may be causing four out of five U.S. asthma-related deaths per year and should be taken off the market, researchers from Cornell and Stanford universities have concluded after a search of medical literature." ("Common asthma inhalers cause up to 80 percent of asthma-related deaths, Cornell and Stanford researchers assert. Cornell Chronicle. March 21, 2017. By Krishna Ramanujan 38)

The U.S. Government has known for 40 years that substances in Cannabis could treat asthma. Yet, they have refused to reschedule it, which hinders research. Many of these 250,000 deaths were children, killed by the medication their government deemed to be safe. The ability to make a safer medication from Cannabis for asthma has been continuously delayed because of current law.

2. Anticonvulsant

There are an estimated 50,000 deaths from epilepsy each year. Many take multiple medications, without any relief. The majority of people who die from epilepsy are those who have the most seizures. Cannabis oil has proven to relieve these seizures in some people (either thc-a oil, or cbd oil, depending on the type of epilepsy.) The prescription medications given for epilepsy can have severe side effects, and in some cases are debilitating.

The inability to create, and test, a drug from Cannabis to treat epilepsy possibly results in thousands of deaths each year. The National Institute of Drug Abuse admitted that Cannabis could possibly treat this disease in 1975—and there was no follow-up.

3. Analgesia

Opiate pain killers—and other opiates—caused 21,000 deaths last year, and countless deaths since the 1970's, when NIDA's report was released. Because opiates are physically addicting, many begin with prescription pain killers, but end up on heroin. The U.S. Government knew in 1977 that Cannabis is an effective pain killer, without the risk of overdose. Instead of rescheduling this drug, so research could be performed—they made opiates more readily available to the population, and are therefore partially to blame for the current opioid epidemic.

4. Antidepressant

Antidepressant overdoses are the second cause of deaths from all drug overdoses. No one has ever died from a Marijuana overdose, yet our government has approved many antidepressants that are dangerous, in many ways. Sudden withdrawal from these medications can cause delusions leading to violence, and some medications themselves can lead to suicide:

> "Antidepressants can raise the risk of suicide, the biggest ever review has found, as pharmaceutical companies were accused of failing to report side-effects and even deaths linked to the drugs. An analysis of 70 trials of the most common antidepressants - involving more than 18,000 people - found they doubled the risk of suicide and aggressive behaviour in under 18s. Although a similarly stark link was not seen in adults, the authors said misreporting of trial data could have led to a 'serious under-estimation of the harms.'" (Antidepressants can raise the risk of suicide, biggest ever review finds. The Telegraph By Sarah Knapton, Science Editor. January 27, 2016 39)

Many of these people who committed suicide were teenagers, and young adults. Our government has approved these drugs to treat depression, but research into a drug from Cannabis to treat depression has not been performed since its antidepressant properties were recognized NIDA's 1977 report. Since that time, countless people have taken these drugs, and many have ended their lives in suicide. Current law constrains research into a drug made from Cannabis that has no psychoactive effects, and lacks the dangerous side effects of current antidepressant medications.

5. Treatment of Alcohol and Drug Dependence

As stated, 20,000 people die each year from alcohol overdose. In the 1977 report to Congress, we read that marijuana could be used in the treatment of alcoholism, and drug dependence. Instead, many in government embraced in a "gateway drug" theory, erroneously believing that Cannabis does "something to the brain" that makes people crave other drugs. In NIDA's report, we discover the opposite. And, the fact that opiate deaths have fallen in every State that has approved medical marijuana laws, prove NIDA's observations were correct. This was a rare time in their history, where truth prevailed over government propaganda.

NIDA also reported in 1977 that Cannabis has anti-tumor effects. Despite this report, the United States Government has continued to place marijuana in the strictest category, a declaration of no medicinal value. This decision has led to a man's death, who suffered from grape-fruit sized tumors protruding throughout his body. Cannabis oil reduced the size of these tumors, and kept this man alive. Before he was sentenced, he stated that a conviction would lead to his death:

"A dying man who claims he grew marijuana to treat a painful cancer faces a possible prison sentence after a conviction on drug charges Wednesday — a prospect he views as a "death sentence. Scott County jurors delivered a guilty verdict on four felony drug charges facing Benton Mackenzie, 48, whose wife and son were also convicted alongside him. Mackenzie says he used the plants to extract cannabis oil to treat a painful grapefruit-sized tumor on his buttock caused by angiosarcoma, a rare, aggressive cancer." (USA Today, Cancer patient says pot conviction a 'death sentence' July 10, 2014 40)

Since neither the United States Government, or the State of Iowa, recognized the medicinal properties of marijuana, the judge would not allow a medical necessity defense. It was not long however, until this man died of his disease while on probation, unable to use marijuana:

"Even as he faced his final moments, Benton Mackenzie's first thoughts were of his wife and son and their future. The 49-year-old terminal cancer patient who fought Scott County authorities over his efforts to grow marijuana for his own medicinal use died early Monday at home....As Mackenzie stood trial, his health deteriorated. The baggy sweatpants he wore masked huge cancerous tumors covering his rear and right leg, a symptom of the angiosarcoma he was diagnosed with in 2011. He was rushed to an emergency room in the middle of his trial for a blood transfusion. Jurors were not allowed to hear any testimony about his health and convicted him along with Loretta for conspiring to grow marijuana.

Their son, Cody, was convicted of drug possession. They all were sentenced to probation in September, and as his rare cancer progressed into the final stages, Benton Mackenzie spent the remaining months of 2014 mostly confined to a hospice bed at his parents' basement apartment in Long Grove." (Family of Benton Mackenzie mourns his death . The Quad City Times. By Brian Wellner. Jan 13, 2015)

While on probation, he was not allowed to use Cannabis oil, so he died. He died suffering, of huge tumors growing out of his body. Consider this news report, in light of NIDA's report in 1977. Back then—four decades ago—our government knew that marijuana had anti-tumor effects. However, instead of funding research, the government continued prohibition. This prohibition took away the right of this man to treat his disease, and he died because of it.

Yet, this is merely one man who suffered and died. The list of deaths caused by these laws could be astronomical. 390,000 Cancer deaths; 20,000 Alcohol overdose deaths; 250,000 Asthma deaths; 21,000 opiate deaths, and 50,000 death from seizures. This means that each year, it is possible that 731,000 die indirectly due to Cannabis prohibition.

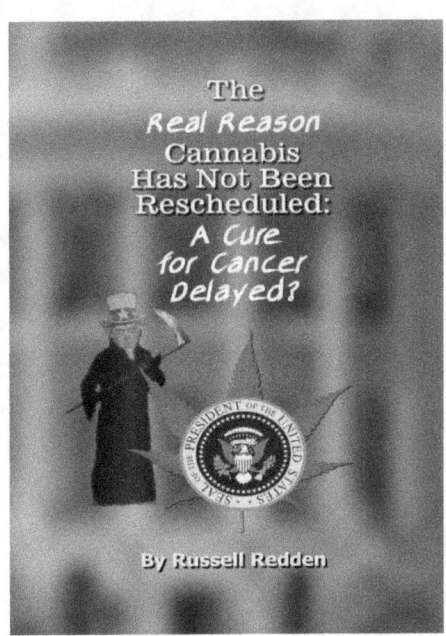

What you don't know...
Can Hurt Everyone!

Richard Nixon and the 91st Congress created a "Catch-22" in the Controlled Substances Act that makes rescheduling Marijuana *next to impossible*.
At the same time, over 100 pre-clinical Studies—performed since 1974—indicate that substances in Cannabis can kill cancer cells.
Yet, our government remains *uninterested*.

This book approaches this subject in a different way. It is designed to argue common sense to the most well educated skeptic. Instead of presenting this evidence as "proof" that marijuana "cures cancer"—it presents this evidence as proof that studies should have been performed on human beings *decades ago*. It compares the government ignoring this issue to the amount of tax dollars spent on other possible cures for cancer, while this one is *ignored*. This book attempts to connect on an emotional level, as well as intellectual, while steering clear of conspiracy theories, and data that is too technical. It presents news stories, and over 100 abstracts as evidence, and compares this evidence to the inaction of the United States government, while people continue to die of these diseases.

Everyone should understand this possible cancer cure, because *we cannot wait* on our government to test it, and make it available. Everyone should also understand what needs to be done in order to make United States drug laws comply with the rights given to us under the U.S. Constitution.

Available on Amazon and Kindle
www.cureforcancerdelayed.com

www.ingramcontent.com/pod-product-compliance
Lightning Source LLC
Chambersburg PA
CBHW061227180526
45170CB00003B/1185